Miracles in Pregnancy

Faith-Fueled Strategies & Prayers for Expectant Moms

Miracles in Pregnancy

Faith-Fueled Strategies & Prayers for Expectant Moms

KIMONA HANSON

Copyright © 2024 Kimona Hanson

ISBN **979-8-9917314-0-9**

All rights reserved. No part of this publication may be reproduced, distributed, or transmitted in any form or by any means, including photocopying, recording, or other electronic or mechanical methods, without the prior written permission of the publisher, except in the case of brief quotations embodied in critical reviews and specific other noncommercial uses permitted by copyright law. All Scriptures were used from the Public Domain.

All scriptures are taken from the NIV Public Domain.

For permission requests, write to the publisher, addressed "Attention: Permissions Coordinator," at the email address below.

Special pricing is available on quantity purchases by corporations, associations, and others. For details, contact the publisher at the email address below.

Orders by U.S. trade bookstores and wholesalers.
Contact Kimona Hanson at kimonahanson@hotmail.com

Printed in the United States of America

Publisher: Kimona Hanson
Publisher Consultant

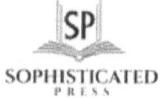

SOPHISTICATED
PRESS

Table of Contents

Introduction – My Story 1

Chapter 1 – Soaked in Prayer 10

Chapter 2 – Healthy Eating and Taking Care of Yourself 16

Chapter 3 – Working 20

Chapter 4 – God's Miracle at 38 23

Chapter 5 – The Power of God's Word During Your Pregnancy 27

Chapter 6 – Daily Declarations 31

Chapter 7 – Generational Blessings 36

Chapter 8 – Living Life for God 38

Bonus – Music List 40

About The Author 42

INTRODUCTION
My Story

As I sit down to write this book, I am filled with gratitude for the journey that has led me here. My pregnancy journey has been one of the most humbling experiences of my life, and it has taught me so much about the power of prayer and faith. My journey began when I married my wonderful husband, whom I believe was God-ordained for me. I remember the day we met vividly. I was on the bus, and a handsome dark chocolate man joined the bus I was riding in. The first thought that crossed my mind was that he would be my husband. I don't know why I felt that way, but I did. I noticed he wore the same work T-shirt as me, which said "Healthfirst." My heart was flustered as I realized we both worked for the same company. I was ecstatic, scared, and terrified all at the same time. I don't even think he noticed me. The stop came, and he got off. I said a short prayer to God while I was still on the bus, "I said Lord, if it is your will, please let us meet again, Amen."

About two weeks later, I was meeting with a couple of friends at a company meeting. I turned around, and guess who I saw? The same guy who was on the bus ride with me. We immediately locked eyes. It was like he knew me already, and I knew him. After the meeting, he approached me, and the first thing he said to me was, "Are you from Ghana? Are you a Ghanaian woman?" I said yes, and yes. He was so happy to hear that and said I'm also Ghanaian. We hit it off immediately, and he gave me his business card. I put it in my pocket, and I thought about him frequently. During that period, I was in a relationship, the person I was dating didn't align with my husbandly ideals. Despite this, I exercised prudence, refraining from hastiness to prevent any emotional harm. My aim was to conscientiously conclude the relationship before embarking on a new chapter.

Shortly after, I remember going out with a few friends, and we talked about our relationship issues and all the bad things happening in our relationships. I was telling them how bad this relationship was that I was in, and I needed to get out. My friend said, "Yeah, you need to move on. You're beautiful, you're smart, and you deserve better." I remember her saying, "I know this guy in this company. When I spoke to him, I thought about you, and I think you guys will be such a great couple." I said, "Who is this guy?" She described the guy, who was the same guy from the bus who introduced himself to me at the meeting. It immediately dawned on me that this might be fate. This might be destiny. I came to this conclusion because my friend mentioned him, and he approached me with his business card. Now a month has passed since he gave me his business card.

Three months later, I was home one day, thinking about him, and I was like, you know what, let me call him. So, I called him, and he picked up, and I said, "Hello, it's Kimona," I said. He responded, saying, "I'm truly grateful for your call." From that moment on, we talked on the phone daily for hours. It was never a day that went by that we didn't talk. From then on, we immediately decided to consummate our relationship and became a couple. Within two years, we got married, and that's how I met my husband.

My journey began when I got married. Shortly after my wedding, I got pregnant with our first child. I was excited and couldn't wait to hold my little one. When I found out, I immediately shared the news with my husband, who was just as thrilled. As my pregnancy progressed, I experienced all the typical symptoms of morning sickness, fatigue, and back pain. However, in my excitement, I neglected to properly care for myself during my pregnancy.

I ignored what I was eating, and I didn't exercise. I constantly worried about the baby's health, which increased my stress. As a result of my poor habits, I ended up having a traumatic C-section delivery. It was a long and painful labor, but eventually, our beautiful baby girl was born, and we were both overwhelmed with love and joy. Navigating the early days of parenthood filled us with uncertainty, especially when it came to caring for our newborn. However, with invaluable presence of my grandmother from Ghana and the support of my mom, we quickly adapted to the responsibilities and established comforting routines. Their guidance made the transition to caring for a newborn much smoother, turning what could have been a stressful experience into a manageable one.

Recovering from a C-section entails a significant physical and emotional journey, and the environment and emotional support you have play crucial roles in the speed of your recovery. During my postpartum period, I adhered to a routine that contributed immensely to my swift healing.

My postpartum routine consisted of several key elements. Firstly, ensuring a tranquil and supportive environment at home was paramount. This involved creating a serene space that promoted relaxation and aided in reducing stress levels. Emotional support, both from my partner and close family members, was integral. Their encouragement and assistance provided a comforting atmosphere, which proved instrumental in my recovery.

In terms of physical care, maintaining a well-balanced diet rich in nutrients was vital. Adequate hydration and a focus on nourishing foods were essential components. Gentle exercises, as recommended by my healthcare provider, played a vital role in gradually restoring my strength without exerting undue stress.

Ensuring sufficient rest was another crucial aspect of my routine. Establishing a consistent sleep schedule, taking short naps when possible, and delegating responsibilities to supportive family members allowed me to prioritize rest, a key factor in the recovery process.

Additionally, incorporating mindfulness practices such as deep breathing exercises and moments of reflection contributed to the overall well-being of body and mind. This routine, though personalized to my needs, can serve as a general guide for anyone navigating the postpartum period, emphasizing the importance of a supportive environment, balanced nutrition, gentle exercise, ample rest, and mindfulness practices.

After a three-year break, I consciously decided to take better care of myself in preparation for my second pregnancy. I was determined to do things differently the next time around.

One significant change involved integrating exercise into my daily routine, consuming nutritious shakes, and embracing a mindful approach to eating. My objective was to defy the concept of "eating for two" and instead concentrate on nourishing my body harmoniously. I committed to a healthy diet, engaged in daily workouts, maintained a regular prayer practice, and recited affirmations related to my pregnancy each day.

As a believer, my approach to mindful eating was characterized by:

- Viewing food as a gift from God. I approached each meal with reverence, grateful for the sustenance it provided for both me and my unborn child.

- Each bite was an opportunity to be fully present, recognizing that God's grace was manifesting through the flavors and textures that nourished my body.

- By listening to my inner signals of hunger and satisfaction, I honored the wisdom that the Creator had instilled within me.

- Before each meal, I offered prayers of gratitude, acknowledging the abundant blessings and sustenance bestowed upon me.

- Mindful eating reaffirmed my trust in God's plan for both my pregnancy and overall well-being. It was a way of aligning my choices with His divine intention.

- Mindful eating taught me humility, encouraging me to approach food with moderation and appreciation, honoring the balance that God has designed.

- This approach wasn't solely about nourishing the body; it was about nurturing my soul's connection with the act of eating, seeing it as an opportunity for spiritual communion.

By weaving faith into my mindful eating journey, I experienced not only physical well-being but also a profound sense of spiritual alignment, recognizing God's presence in every nourishing bite.

As I embarked on my 2nd pregnancy journey, I encountered skepticism from doctors regarding the possibility of a vaginal birth after a cesarean (VBAC). They emphasized the statistical likelihood of having another C-section. However, I chose to put my faith in God rather than accepting their pessimistic outlook. I firmly believed that God had promised me a healthy and successful delivery, and I held onto that promise through unwavering faith and prayer.

Though I faced challenges along the way, I never wavered in my trust in God's plan for me. I knew that challenges are a part of any journey, but it was my faith that anchored me through them. My faith allowed me to approach my second pregnancy differently, with a newfound sense of confidence and determination.

Despite being told that a vaginal birth would be difficult due to my previous C-section, I refused to give up hope. With God's help, I was able to have a natural birth, defying all odds and expectations. Ultimately, my faith was vindicated. Despite unfavorable odds, I had VBAC (Vaginal Birth After Cesarean), surpassing the predictions of medical experts. This accomplishment underscored the potency of faith and the resilience that arises from placing my trust in God.

I am thrilled to share the joyous news of the arrival of my vibrant baby boy, Levi. It was indescribable when I heard my baby's cry for the first time. It was like music to my ears, and my heart was filled with an overwhelming sense of joy and gratitude. I felt like I had accomplished something incredible, and it was all thanks to God's grace and help. It was a moment I would never forget. It made all the hard work, sacrifice, and determination worth it. Seeing my baby's little face for the first time, holding him in my arms, and feeling his warm skin against mine was truly magical. It was a reminder that anything is possible with faith, perseverance, and determination.

As I pondered about my second pregnancy journey, I've come to recognize the profound influence that my thoughts, belief structure, and faith wielded over my experience during my pregnancy. It became evident that my actions and daily activities also played a significant role in having a successful pregnancy experience. By placing my complete trust in God, praying fervently, and surrendering control, I allowed God's guidance to shape my journey. I consciously decided to do things differently than I did during my first pregnancy. It was a complete transformation from my previous approach, resulting in a beautiful testimony.

My mindset and belief system were vital in shaping my pregnancy experience. Embracing positive thoughts, affirmations, and a deep-rooted faith enabled me to navigate the challenges with grace and strength. I discovered the power of aligning my actions with my faith, knowing that God's promises never fail.

Every step of the way, I felt His presence guiding and protecting me. It was an incredible testament to the miracles that unfold when we surrender our worries and fears to God. Through the trials and triumphs, I witnessed firsthand the profound impact that faith can have on our lives. I share this experience to inspire others to trust in God's plan, to believe in the power of positive thinking, and to embrace a faith-driven approach to their journeys. May my testimony serve as a reminder that no matter the challenges we face, with God at the helm, we can overcome and emerge with a beautiful and awe-inspiring story.

As I embark on this new chapter of motherhood, I am filled with gratitude for the faith that carried me through and the blessings that have come my way. May your journey be blessed with abundant joy, unwavering faith, and the strength to embrace each moment with grace.

Through each pregnancy, I learned that prayer and faith are essential tools in navigating the challenges of motherhood. It is not always easy, and there were times when I wanted to give up, but I knew that God was always with me, providing me with strength, courage, and wisdom.

I want to share my experiences and lessons with other mothers-to-be. Pregnancy can be overwhelming and uncertain, but with prayer and faith, we can find peace and strength to overcome any obstacle. This book is for every mother who wants to connect with God and find the courage and wisdom to navigate the challenges of pregnancy and motherhood. It will serve as a guide and inspiration for all mothers-to-be. May it be a reminder that no matter how challenging the journey may be, with faith and prayer, anything is possible.

Here are 15 things I did to change the course of my last two pregnancies:

1. I ate healthy: I ate a balanced diet with plenty of fruits, vegetables, and lean protein.

2. I exercised: I walked regularly and did prenatal yoga to stay active and healthy.

3. I prayed: I made a daily habit of praying for my baby's health and my well-being.

4. I thought positively: I focused on the joy and excitement of pregnancy rather than the fear and uncertainty.

5. I trusted my body: I believed that my body could deliver a baby naturally, despite having a C-section with my first child.

6. I surrounded myself with positivity. I sought support from friends, family, and other expectant mothers with similar goals and beliefs.

7. I stayed informed: I did my research on natural childbirth and sought out resources that could help me prepare for the delivery.

8. I trusted my instincts: I listened to my body and followed my intuition, even when it went against conventional wisdom.

9. I sought a supportive healthcare provider. I found a doctor who respected my wishes and supported my desire for a natural birth.

10. I stayed focused on my goal. I kept my eye on the prize and never lost sight of my desire for a natural, healthy birth.

11. I prayed daily for strength, courage, and wisdom throughout my pregnancy.

12. I fasted for a few hours daily, seeking God's guidance and favor on my pregnancy journey.

13. I made daily confessions for myself and my baby, declaring health, safety, and smooth delivery.

14. I visualized a successful delivery and healthy baby, using the power of my mind to manifest a positive outcome.

15. I trusted in God's plan for me and my baby, surrendering my fears and anxieties to Him and embracing faith over fear.

Through these 15 actions, I was able to change the course of my last two pregnancies. I had successful, natural births that were empowering and transformative experiences. I learned that anything is possible with prayer, faith, and a positive mindset. I hope that by sharing my story and the lessons I've learned along the way, other mothers-to-be will be inspired to trust their bodies, stay positive, and embrace the journey of pregnancy and childbirth with confidence and joy.

CHAPTER 1

Soaked in Prayer

Congratulations on embarking on this incredible journey of pregnancy and parenthood! As you navigate the ups and downs of this season, may you be filled with God's love, hope, and strength.

This book will explore the power of prayer, healthy habits, and God's promises for a healthy pregnancy and generational blessings. As you progress on your pregnancy journey, I encourage you to continue prioritizing your relationship with God and seek His guidance and wisdom.

Prayer is a powerful tool that can help you navigate the challenges and joys of pregnancy. As you prepare to bring new life into the world, it's essential to cultivate a solid spiritual foundation. Here are some ways to do just that.

Create a Prayer Space

One way to make prayer a regular part of your pregnancy routine is to create a designated prayer space in your home. Depending on your preferences, this can be a small corner of a room or a larger area. Decorate the space with items that are meaningful to you, such as religious art, candles, or books. Ensure the space is quiet and free from distractions so that you can focus on your prayers.

Pray for Yourself

It's important to pray for yourself during pregnancy, as well as for your unborn child. Take time each day to ask God for strength, wisdom, and guidance as you navigate this new phase of life. Pray for your health and the health of your baby. Ask God to give you the patience and grace you need to handle any challenges that arise.

Pray for Your Baby

Praying for your baby is a beautiful way to connect with your child before birth. You can pray for your baby's health, safety, and happiness. Ask God to bless your child with a kind heart, a curious mind, and a love for others. You can also pray for your child's future, asking God to guide them in the coming years.

Connect with Other Praying Moms

Connecting with other moms also committed to prayer can be a great source of support and encouragement during pregnancy. Look for local prayer groups or join online communities to connect with moms who share your faith. You can also ask friends or family members to pray for you and your baby. Being soaked in prayer is essential to a healthy pregnancy. Creating a prayer space, praying for yourself and your baby, connecting with other praying moms, and trusting in God's plan can help you navigate the ups and downs of pregnancy with grace and peace.

A List of Daily Prayers for Your Pregnancy Journey

To help you stay connected to God and focused on His promises, here is a list of daily prayers that you can incorporate into your routine:

1. Prayer for a healthy pregnancy: *Dear God, I thank you for this blessing of pregnancy and the miracle of life growing inside me. Please watch over my baby and me and grant us the strength and health we need to make it through*

this journey. Please guide my healthcare providers in providing me with the best possible care and help me be proactive in caring for myself and my baby.

2. **Prayer for strength and energy:** *Lord, I ask for your help getting through each day of this pregnancy. Please give me the physical and emotional strength I need to take care of myself and my family and the energy to face any challenges that come my way. Please help me to find moments of rest and relaxation amidst the demands of pregnancy and motherhood.*

3. **Prayer for peace of mind:** *God, I pray for peace of mind during this time of uncertainty and change. Please help me trust in your plan for my life and my child's life and to find comfort in your loving presence. Ease any worries or anxieties I may have and grant me the serenity to enjoy this special time.*

4. **Prayer for wisdom and guidance:** *Heavenly Father, please grant me the wisdom and guidance I need to make informed decisions about my health and my baby's health. Please help me to seek out the resources and support I need to make the best choices for my family and to be proactive in advocating for our well-being. Please guide me in choosing a care provider and birth plan that aligns with my values and goals for this pregnancy and beyond.*

5. **Prayer for a strong bond with my baby:** *Lord, I pray for a deep and lasting bond with my baby during this pregnancy. Please help me to connect with my child in meaningful ways, such as through music, reading, or quiet moments of reflection. Give me the patience and presence to be fully present with my baby and to create a nurturing and loving environment that will support our relationship for years to come.*

6. **Prayer for a healthy environment:** *God, I ask for your guidance in creating a healthy and safe environment for myself and my baby during this pregnancy. Help me to make wise choices about the food I eat, the products I use, and the activities I engage in. Grant me the wisdom to discern what is best for us and the discipline to follow through with healthy habits and routines.*

7. Prayer for a positive attitude: *Lord, please help me to maintain a positive attitude during this pregnancy, even in the midst of challenges and discomfort. Help me to focus on the joy and wonder of bringing new life into the world and to find gratitude in the small moments of each day. Please give me the strength to face any obstacles with grace, resilience, and the humility to ask for help when needed.*

8. Prayer for a healthy community: *God, I pray for a healthy support community during this pregnancy. Help me to connect with other expectant parents, healthcare providers, and spiritual mentors who can offer guidance, encouragement, and friendship. Grant me the courage to be vulnerable and open and the generosity to share my experiences.*

9. Prayer for a safe and healthy world: *Lord, please protect my baby and all babies worldwide from harm and danger. Please help us create a safe and healthy world for all children to grow and thrive. Give me the strength to advocate for the health and well-being of all families and the compassion to extend love and support to those struggling.*

10. Prayer for gratitude: *God, I am grateful for the gift of life and the opportunity to bring new life into the world. Thank you for the gift of life, the miracle of pregnancy, and the joy and love that come with motherhood. I am grateful for the strength and health you have given me and for the support of my loved ones during this journey. Help me to remember your grace and goodness every day and to never take these blessings for granted. As I continue on this pregnancy journey, may my heart overflow with gratitude and praise for all that you have done and continue to do in my life. In Jesus' name, I pray, Amen.*

May these prayers serve as a source of comfort, hope, and strength as you continue on your pregnancy journey. Remember that God loves you and your baby and is always with you, guiding you and providing for you every step of the way.

Here are ten confessions you can make during your pregnancy journey:

1. I confess that I trust God's plan for me and my baby and surrender all my fears and worries to Him.

2. I confess that I will care for my body by eating healthily, exercising, and resting well.

3. I will surround myself with positive and supportive people who will encourage and uplift me during this journey.

4. I confess that I will not let fear or anxiety control my thoughts and emotions, but instead, I will focus on God's peace and love.

5. I confess that I will be patient and kind to myself during this journey, knowing that my body is doing miraculous work of creating life.

6. I confess that I will pray for my baby's health and well-being and teach him/her to love and serve God.

7. I confess that I will speak life and blessings over my baby and not let negative words or thoughts affect him/her.

8. I confess that I will seek wisdom and guidance from God and others who have gone through this journey before me.

9. I confess that I will take time to rest and relax, knowing that it is essential for my baby's and my health.

10. I confess that I will give thanks to God every day for this precious gift of life and His constant love and provision.

I declare that I will have a deep and meaningful connection with my baby from the moment of conception.

1. I declare that my baby will be filled with love, joy, and happiness.

2. I declare that I will have a strong and healthy body throughout my pregnancy.

3. I declare that I will have a positive and empowering birth experience.

4. I declare that my pregnancy journey will be a time of growth, transformation, and blessings.

We will speak more about declarations in Chapter 6.

CHAPTER 2

Healthy Eating and Taking Care of Yourself

Pregnancy is a time of significant physical and emotional changes. It's essential to take care of yourself during this time, not only for your well-being but also for the health of your growing baby. One of the best ways to do this is by adopting healthy eating habits.

Healthy Eating During Pregnancy

Eating a well-balanced diet is essential during pregnancy. Your body needs more nutrients to support the growth and development of your baby. It would be best if you aimed to eat a variety of foods from all the food groups, including:

- Fruits and vegetables: These are a great source of vitamins, minerals, and fiber. Aim to eat at least five servings per day.

- Whole grains: These provide important nutrients such as iron, B vitamins, and fiber. Choose whole-grain bread, rice, and pasta.

- Lean protein: This includes chicken, fish, beans, and tofu. These foods provide essential nutrients such as iron, zinc, and omega-3 fatty acids.

- Dairy products: These are a good source of calcium, which is important for your baby's bones and teeth. Choose low-fat or fat-free options.

Here's a list of nutritious foods that I recommend for pregnant women:

1. Leafy Greens: Spinach, Kale, Swiss Chard, and other leafy greens are rich in essential nutrients like folate, iron, and calcium.

2. Legumes: Lentils, chickpeas, black beans, and other legumes provide a good source of protein, fiber, and folate.

3. Lean Proteins: Opt for lean sources of protein such as poultry, fish (low in mercury), tofu, eggs, and lean cuts of beef or pork.

4. Colorful Fruits: Enjoy a variety of fruits like berries, citrus fruits, apples, pears, and melons, which are packed with vitamins, fiber, and antioxidants.

5. Whole Grains: Include whole grains such as quinoa, brown rice, oats, whole wheat bread, and whole grain pasta for fiber, energy, and important nutrients.

6. Dairy Products: Incorporate sources of calcium, like milk, yogurt, cheese, and fortified plant-based alternatives (if you're lactose intolerant or follow a vegan diet).

7. Healthy Fats: Include sources of healthy fats like avocados, nuts, seeds, and olive oil, which provide omega-3 fatty acids and support fetal development.

8. Colorful Vegetables: Add a variety of vegetables to your plate, including carrots, bell peppers, sweet potatoes, broccoli, and tomatoes, to obtain essential vitamins and minerals.

9. Fortified Foods: Incorporate foods fortified with essential nutrients like iron, such as fortified cereals and bread, to meet increased nutritional needs.

10. Plenty of Water: Stay well-hydrated by drinking adequate water throughout the day. Aim for at least 8-10 cups per day.

Remember to consult your healthcare provider or a registered dietitian for personalized dietary recommendations during pregnancy, as individual needs may vary. Avoid sugary drinks and limit your intake of caffeine.

Managing Nausea and Other Pregnancy Symptoms

Many women experience nausea and other symptoms during pregnancy, especially in the first trimester. Here are some tips for managing these symptoms:

- Eat small, frequent meals throughout the day.

- Avoid foods that are high in fat or spicy.

- Drink ginger tea or ginger ale to help settle your stomach.

- Get plenty of rest and avoid stressful situations.

Exercise During Pregnancy

Exercise is essential during pregnancy, but you should always talk to your doctor before starting any new exercise program. Some good options for pregnant women include:

- Walking: This is a low-impact exercise that is easy to do and can be done almost anywhere.

- Swimming: This is a great way to get a full-body workout without putting stress on your joints.

- Prenatal massages: This can help improve flexibility and strength and provide relaxation and stress relief.

It's important to listen to your body and not overdo it. Avoid activities that are high-impact or involve much jumping or twisting. In conclusion, adopting healthy eating habits and taking care of yourself during pregnancy is essential for your well-being and the health of your growing baby. Eating a well-balanced diet, managing nausea and other symptoms, and getting regular exercise can help you have a healthy pregnancy and prepare you for the joys of motherhood.

CHAPTER 3

Working

During my pregnancies, I continued to work in my role as the Associate Director of Emergency Management Services in the ED. Fortunately, I had a supportive boss, Ms. Vivien Salmon, who was very considerate of my pregnancy. She ensured that I wasn't given any strenuous work and didn't have to do any rounds.

As my pregnancy progressed, Ms. Salmon became even more protective of me. She often suggested that I go home early, worried I might go into labor at work. I appreciated her concern and thoughtfulness.

By the time I reached my third trimester, I was very limited in what I could do. I mostly attended meetings and stuck to desk assignments. Ms. Salmon and the rest of the team were understanding and accommodating, and I was grateful for their support during that time.

Overall, I felt fortunate to have had such a positive experience with work and pregnancy. Ms. Salmon and my colleagues were considerate and supportive, significantly impacting my ability to manage both roles.

Balancing work and pregnancy can be challenging, but taking care of yourself and your baby while fulfilling your work responsibilities is important. Here are some tips for working during pregnancy.

Communicate With Your Employer

One of the first things you should do when you find out you're pregnant is to communicate with your employer. Let them know your due date and any plans you have for maternity leave. Discuss any accommodations you may need, such as more frequent breaks, a more comfortable chair, or a change in your work schedule. Be clear about your limitations, and don't be afraid to ask for help.

Take Breaks Often

Taking frequent breaks is essential during pregnancy, especially if you have a job that requires a lot of sitting or standing. Take short breaks every hour to stretch, move around, and stay hydrated. Consider using a pregnancy pillow to support your back or a footrest to reduce swelling. Take a longer break in the middle of the day to rest or take a short nap.

Stay Comfortable

It's important to stay comfortable while you work during pregnancy. Wear comfortable clothes and shoes that fit well and support your growing body. Adjust your workspace if needed to make it more ergonomic and reduce strain on your body. Use a fan or adjust the temperature in your workspace to keep you cool and comfortable.

Know Your Limits

As your pregnancy progresses, it's important to know your limits and not overdo it. Please pay attention to your body and listen to its cues. If you feel tired, take a break or go home early. Be bold and ask for help with tasks that are too physically demanding or stressful. Remember, taking care of yourself and your baby is your top priority.

Working during pregnancy can be challenging, but balancing work and self-care with some adjustments and planning is possible. Communicating with your employer, taking frequent breaks, staying comfortable, and knowing your limits are all essential to maintaining a healthy pregnancy while working.

CHAPTER 4

God's Miracle at 38

In this chapter of my life, nine years after my initial journey, I find myself raising my two children. At 38 years of age, I made the bold decision to have a third child. Despite the odds and the passing years, I never really factored in my age when it came to expanding my family. Instead, I continued to trust in the miracles of the Almighty.

Over the years, I had postponed this decision, immersed in building my career and business. I kept telling myself that I would start a family next year, but as time passed, my husband rightly reminded me that if we were to have a third child, now was the time. At 38, I embarked on this new journey.

I revisited the doctors, who reviewed my pregnancy history, noting a C-section for my first child and a V-back for my second. They cautioned me about the risks associated with being pregnant at 38, with potential illnesses looming. Turning to the wisdom found in the bible, I drew inspiration from the accounts of Hebrew women who exhibited swift and quick birth. Declaring that I, too, would experience a birthing process akin to theirs, I immersed myself in the biblical narratives, reading and meditating on the stories that resonated with the strength and resilience of these women. Every time the doctors shared negative possibilities, I remembered the divine promise and asked myself, "Whose report will I believe, the word of the Lord or the doctors?"

This divine promise aligns with the biblical truth found in Exodus 1:19: "The midwives said to Pharaoh, "Hebrew women are not like Egyptian women; they are vigorous and give birth before the midwives arrive." This was my declaration, and I held fast to the words of the Lord, who had promised that I would give birth like a Hebrew woman.

Throughout this pregnancy, I underwent various tests due to my age, even being assessed for the risk of Down syndrome. But every test was negative and returned with reassuring results. Even when my sugar levels spiked one day during fasting, I persisted.

When the time came to give birth, I returned to the same hospital as my previous delivery. I maintained the same positive mindset, healthy lifestyle, daily affirmations, and a routine of fasting and prayer. Yet, upon arriving at the hospital, I was told they couldn't proceed with a VBAC (vaginal birth after C-section). They deemed me a high risk due to my weight and other factors that didn't align with my healthy lifestyle.

In that moment, I made a firm decision. I asked to be transferred to a hospital where I could give birth naturally. The doctors had cited a multitude of concerns in my chart, almost classifying me as diabetic and susceptible to many comorbidities. I refused to accept those limitations and chose a hospital that aligned with my faith and vision.

With faith as my guiding light, I began to labor. It was a Tuesday night, and by 11 o'clock the following morning, I had given birth to my third child, a baby boy named Legend. To the glory of God, I had achieved another natural birth with no complications and no C-section. This recovery was smooth and swift.

My message to anyone reading this book is that even in your late thirties, you can give birth. Never feel that you are behind, for with God, all things are possible. I stand as a living testament, a sign and wonder, having given birth to three children, two of them naturally, all because I placed my trust in God.

All because I believed that faith, coupled with works, would bring about a testimony that I could share with the world. It's crucial to understand that sometimes people don't realize that while doctors provide valuable medical advice, their words do not define the Word of the Lord. God's promises are imprinted on my heart, and any pregnant woman reading this should be armed with the Word, ready to speak words of encouragement through life's trials, especially during the journey of childbearing.

During my third pregnancy, I relied on specific scriptures to keep my faith strong and my spirits high. The verses I meditated on daily allowed me to lean on the Lord's promises rather than the words of the medical professionals.

Here are the scriptures that sustained me during my 3rd pregnancy:

1. Jeremiah 32:27 (NIV): I am the Lord, the God of all mankind. Is anything too hard for me?

2. Psalm 71:6 (NIV): From birth I have relied on you; you brought me forth from my mother's womb. I will ever praise you.

3. Galatians 6:9 (NIV): Let us not become weary in doing good, for at the proper time we will reap a harvest if we do not give up.

4. Numbers 23:19 (NIV): God is not human, that he should lie, not a human being, that he should change his mind. Does he speak and then not act? Does he promise and not fulfill?

5. Ecclesiastes 3:11 (NIV): He has made everything beautiful in its time. He has also set eternity in the human heart; yet no one can fathom what God has done from beginning to end.

Each of these verses, standing as pillars of strength, provided me with the grace needed for this remarkable journey of motherhood. Alongside prayer, daily Bible reading, maintaining my appearance, walking regularly, and joining a local mom group, my faith remained unwavering as I placed my trust in the Word of the Lord.

CHAPTER 5

The Power of God's Word During Your Pregnancy

The Bible is a powerful tool that can provide comfort, strength, and guidance during pregnancy. Here are some ways to incorporate God's Word into your pregnancy journey.

Read the Bible Daily

Making time to read the Bible daily can help you feel more grounded and connected to God during pregnancy. Choose a time of day that works for you, whether it's in the morning, during your lunch break, or before bed. Use a Bible app or a physical Bible to read a few verses or a chapter daily. You can also use a devotional book or Bible study guide for pregnancy-specific readings and reflections.

Meditate on Scripture

Meditating on Scripture is another way to incorporate God's Word into your pregnancy routine. Choose a verse or passage that speaks to you and reflect on its meaning. Repeat the verse to yourself throughout the day or write it down and carry it with you. You can also create art or crafts inspired by the verse to help you remember its message.

Pray with Scripture

Praying with Scripture is a powerful way to connect with God and ask for His guidance during pregnancy. Choose a verse or passage that speaks to your current situation and use it as a basis for your prayers. You can also use the Bible's prayers and Psalms as a template for your prayers. Consider starting a prayer journal to record your prayers and reflect on God's answers.

Join a Bible Study Group

Joining a Bible study group is a great way to connect with other Christians and deepen your understanding of God's Word. Look for local Bible study groups or join online communities to connect with other moms who share your faith. You can also ask your church or local Christian bookstore for recommendations. A Bible study group can provide accountability, support, and encouragement during pregnancy.

Incorporating God's Word into your pregnancy routine can provide comfort, strength, and guidance during this special time. Reading the Bible daily, meditating on Scripture, praying with Scripture, and joining a Bible study group are all ways to deepen your faith and connect with God's plan for your pregnancy journey.

Here are some Bible scriptures that you can use during pregnancy:

1. Psalm 139:13-14 - "For you created my inmost being; you knit me together in my mother's womb. I praise you because I am fearfully and wonderfully made; your works are wonderful, I know that full well."

2. Isaiah 44:24 - "This is what the LORD says--your Redeemer, who formed you in the womb: I am the LORD, the Maker of all things, who stretches out the heavens, who spread out the earth by myself."

3. Jeremiah 1:5 - "Before I formed you in the womb I knew you, before you were born I set you apart; I appointed you as a prophet to the nations."

4. Luke 1:42 - "In a loud voice she [Elizabeth] exclaimed: 'Blessed are you among women, and blessed is the child you will bear!'"

5. Galatians 1:15 - "But when God, who set me apart from my mother's womb and called me by his grace, was pleased."

6. Psalm 127:3 - "Children are a heritage from the LORD, offspring a reward from him."

7. 1 Samuel 1:27 - "I prayed for this child, and the LORD has granted me what I asked of him."

8. Psalm 22:9-10 - "Yet you brought me out of the womb; you made me trust in you, even at my mother's breast. From birth I was cast on you; from my mother's womb you have been my God."

9. Isaiah 49:1 - "Before I was born the LORD called me; from my mother's womb he has spoken my name."

10. Job 10:10 - "Did you not pour me out like milk and curdle me like cheese?"

11. Psalm 71:6 - "From birth I have relied on you; you brought me forth from my mother's womb. I will ever praise you."

12. Job 31:15 - "Did not he who made me in the womb make them? Did not the same one form us both within our mothers?"

13. Ecclesiastes 11:5 - "As you do not know the path of the wind, or how the body is formed in a mother's womb, so you cannot understand the work of God, the Maker of all things."

14. Luke 1:36 - "Even Elizabeth your relative is going to have a child in her old age, and she who was said to be unable to conceive is in her sixth month."

15. Psalm 113:9 - "He settles the childless woman in her home as a happy mother of children. Praise the LORD."

16. Psalm 128:3 - "Your wife will be like a fruitful vine within your house; your children will be like olive shoots around your table."

17. Isaiah 66:13a - "As a mother comforts her child, so will I [God] comfort you."

18. Genesis 25:21 - "Isaac prayed to the LORD on behalf of his wife, because she was childless. The LORD answered his prayer and his wife Rebekah became pregnant."

19. Exodus 23:26 - "No one will miscarry or be barren in your land, and I will give you a full life span."

20. Proverbs 17:6 - "Children's children are a crown to the aged, and parents are the pride of their children.

CHAPTER 6

Daily Declarations

Daily declarations are a powerful way to speak life and truth over yourself and your baby during pregnancy. Here are some tips for creating and using daily declarations.

What are Daily Declarations?

Daily declarations are positive statements you can repeat to yourself throughout the day to help shift your mindset and focus on God's promises. These statements can be tailored to your specific needs and situation during pregnancy. Examples of daily declarations include "I am strong and capable," "My baby is healthy and growing," and "God is with me always."

How to Create Daily Declarations

Creating daily declarations is a simple process. Start by identifying areas of your life or pregnancy journey where you want positive change or growth. Then, use scripture or other positive affirmations to create statements that speak to those areas. For example, if you're struggling with anxiety, a daily declaration might be, "God has not given me a spirit of fear, but of power, love, and a sound mind" (2 Timothy 1:7).

How to Use Daily Declarations

Using daily declarations is easy and can be done throughout the day. Choose a few declarations that resonate with you and repeat them to yourself several times daily. You can say them out loud or silently to yourself. Consider writing them down and placing them in prominent places around your home or workplace as reminders. You can also create a daily declaration ritual, such as saying them before you get out of bed in the morning or before meals.

Benefits of Daily Declarations

Daily declarations can have many benefits during pregnancy. They can help you shift your focus away from negative thoughts or fears and toward God's promises. They can also help you cultivate a positive mindset and a sense of gratitude. Daily declarations can also provide comfort and encouragement during difficult moments or times of uncertainty.

Daily declarations are positive affirmations you make about yourself and your life regularly. By reciting these affirmations daily, you can empower yourself in several ways:

1. Boosting confidence: Daily declarations can help you build confidence in yourself and your abilities. When you repeatedly affirm positive things about yourself, you start to believe them and internalize them as part of your identity. This can help you approach challenges with a more positive and confident mindset.

2. Reframing negative thoughts: Often, we have negative thoughts or beliefs about ourselves that hold us back. Daily declarations can help you reframe those negative thoughts into positive ones, which can help you overcome limiting beliefs and achieve your goals.

3. Fostering a growth mindset: By focusing on positive affirmations, you can cultivate a growth mindset, believing that your abilities and

intelligence can be developed through dedication and hard work. This can help you stay motivated and persistent in the face of obstacles.

4. Improving mood and well-being: Reciting positive affirmations can help improve your mood and overall well-being. Focusing on positive thoughts and emotions makes you more likely to experience feelings of happiness, gratitude, and contentment.

Daily declarations are a simple and powerful way to speak the truth and live over yourself and your baby during pregnancy. Creating and using daily declarations can help you focus on God's promises and cultivate a positive mindset. Consider incorporating daily declarations into your pregnancy routine for added peace and encouragement.

Here are the daily declarations that I used during your pregnancy journey:

1. I declare that my pregnancy will be a healthy and joyful experience.

2. I declare that my baby will be born strong, healthy, and perfect in every way.

3. I declare that I will have a safe and smooth delivery.

4. I declare that I will have an abundance of energy and strength throughout my pregnancy.

5. I declare and decree that my pregnancy is blessed by God and will bring forth a healthy and happy baby.

6. I declare that my body is strong and capable of carrying my baby to full term.

7. I declare that God fearfully and wonderfully made my baby, and I will cherish and love him/her unconditionally.

8. I declare that I will use this time to deepen my relationship with God and trust in His promises for me and my baby.

9. I declare that my labor and delivery will be safe and smooth, and I will quickly recover.

10. I declare I will have a peaceful and calm mind during my pregnancy.

11. I declare that I will have a deep and restful sleep every night.

12. I declare that my baby will grow and develop according to God's perfect plan.

13. I declare that I will have a strong and healthy immune system to protect my baby.

14. I declare that I will have a strong and healthy emotional well-being during my pregnancy.

15. I declare that I will have a healthy and balanced diet that nourishes both me and my baby.

16. I declare that I will have a strong and healthy connection with my partner and family during my pregnancy.

17. I declare that I will have a strong and healthy bond with my baby.

18. I declare that I will have a positive and optimistic outlook on my pregnancy journey.

19. I declare that I will have a strong and healthy support system during my pregnancy.

20. I declare that I will have a strong and healthy spiritual connection during my pregnancy.

21. I declare that I will have a deep and meaningful connection with my baby from the moment of conception.

22. I declare that my baby will be filled with love, joy, and happiness.

23. I declare that I will have a strong and healthy body throughout my pregnancy.

24. I declare that I will have a positive and empowering birth experience.

CHAPTER 7

Generational Blessings

As a parent, you can pass down generational blessings to your children. Here are some ways to intentionally create a legacy of blessings for your family.

Praying for children

One of the most powerful ways to bless your children is through prayer. Pray for their health, safety, and well-being. Pray for their relationships and future. Pray for their spiritual growth and development. Consistent prayer can profoundly impact your children's lives and future generations.

Speak Blessings Over Your Children

In addition to prayer, speaking blessings over your children is another way to create a legacy of generational blessings. This can be done through daily declarations (as discussed in Chapter 5) or through intentional conversations with your children. Speak words of affirmation and encouragement over them. Tell them how much you love and appreciate them. Remind them of their God-given identity and purpose.

Live a Life of Faith

Your life can be a powerful example to your children and future generations. Live a life of faith and obedience to God's Word. Demonstrate the fruit of the Spirit (love, joy, peace, patience, kindness, goodness, faithfulness, gentleness, and self-control) in your actions and interactions with others. Show your children what it means to trust in God and follow His plan for your life.

Pass Down Family Traditions

Family traditions can be a meaningful way to pass down generational blessings. Create traditions that center around your faith and values. For example, you might have a family Bible study or prayer time each week or celebrate certain holidays or milestones in ways that honor God. These traditions can create a sense of connection and continuity between generations.

Creating a legacy of generational blessings is a powerful way to impact your family and future generations. Praying for your children, speaking blessings over them, living a life of faith, and passing down family traditions are all ways to create a legacy of blessings intentionally. Consider incorporating these practices into your family life to leave a lasting impact on your children and future generations.

CHAPTER 8

Living Life for God

As you journey through pregnancy and parenthood, it's important to remember that every aspect of your life can be lived for God's glory. Here are some ways to prioritize your relationship with God and honor Him in every area of your life.

Prioritize Time with God

Make time for God a priority in your daily routine. Set aside time daily to pray, read the Bible, or engage in other spiritual practices that help you connect with God. Consider waking up a little earlier or setting aside time before bed to spend with God. When you make time for God, you'll find He is faithful to meet you and fill you with His presence and peace.

Serve Others with Love

Jesus calls us to love and serve others; pregnancy and parenthood provide many opportunities. Look for ways to help those around you, whether volunteering, supporting a friend in need, or simply offering a kind word or gesture. You'll find your heart filled with joy and gratitude as you serve others with love.

Practice Gratitude

Gratitude is a powerful spiritual practice that can transform your perspective and help you live life for God's glory. Take time each day to reflect on the blessings in your life, both big and small. Express gratitude to God and those around you for the gifts and blessings you've received. When you live with a heart of gratitude, you'll find that your perspective shifts and your joy and contentment increase.

Live with Purpose

God has a unique purpose for your life; pregnancy and parenthood allow you to discover and live out that purpose. Consider what gifts and talents God has given you and how you can use them to serve Him and others. Seek out opportunities to live with purpose, whether it's through your work, your relationships, or your community involvement. When you live purposefully, you'll find your life meaningful and significant.

Living life for God is a powerful way to honor Him and find fulfillment and joy in every season of life, including pregnancy and parenthood. Prioritizing time with God, serving others with love, practicing gratitude, and living purposefully are just a few ways to live for God's glory. May you be inspired to live every aspect of your life for Him and find abundant blessings and joy as you do.

BONUS

Music List

Here is my playlist that I listened to during my pregnancy and after that is filled with uplifting songs that will inspire and uplift your spirits:

1. "Good Grace" by Hillsong UNITED
2. "Oceans (Where Feet May Fail)" by Hillsong UNITED
3. "Way Maker" by Sinach
4. "Reckless Love" by Cory Asbury
5. "Great Are You Lord" by All Sons & Daughters
6. "10,000 Reasons (Bless the Lord)" by Matt Redman
7. "What a Beautiful Name" by Hillsong Worship
8. "Build My Life" by Housefires
9. "King of My Heart" by Bethel Music
10. "I Can Only Imagine" by Mercy Me
11. "You Say" by Lauren Daigle
12. "Who You Say I Am" by Hillsong Worship
13. "No Longer Slaves" by Bethel Music
14. "How He Loves" by David Crowder Band

15. "The Stand" by Hillsong UNITED

These songs carry messages of faith, hope, and the power of God's love. They are perfect for uplifting your spirits, encouraging reflection, and strengthening your faith during pregnancy.

About The Author

Kimona Hanson is an author and faith-based entrepreneur who believes in the power of faith, perseverance, and the guiding hand of God. With a deep conviction in the importance of aligning one's life with spiritual principles, Kimona Hanson shares her personal journey and experiences as an expectant mother in her book. Drawing from her challenges, triumphs, and unwavering faith, she offers insights, strategies, and inspiration to empower other women on their paths of pregnancy and motherhood. Through her writing, Kimona aims to uplift, encourage, and guide readers to embrace the divine guidance available to them, ensuring a fulfilling and faith-filled journey.

www.ingramcontent.com/pod-product-compliance
Lightning Source LLC
Chambersburg PA
CBHW051949160426
43198CB00013B/2366